A Year of Positive Thinking

An Inspiration For Each Day of the Year

By: CONNIE CONNIE ROSCOE

TABLE OF CONTENTS

INTRODUCTION

Positive thinking along with gratitude, brings you not only success but in your daily life it also brings you inner peace, improved relationships, better health, happiness and joy. It also helps you to look at life with a whole new meaning... your daily affairs will run more smoothly, life will actually look brighter and even promising.

Positive thinking is also contagious just like a smile or laughter! Think about it - have you ever been with someone who is laughing at a joke or something funny that happened, and they can't stop laughing? Then, as they finally are able to control their laughter, they are thinking about the joke or funny incident and start laughing again... it makes you laugh right along with them - you can't help but laugh with them!

People around you will pick up on your positive attitude and are affected accordingly. Think about happy things - remember... for every negative, there is a positive. For every negative thought that comes into your mind, think of something positive about it, for instance... you are at work thinking how much you absolutely hate your job - think about how many thousands of people have lost their jobs over the past couple of years and have not been able to find another one! Now you are thankful (this is where gratitude steps in along with the positive thinking) that you at least HAVE a job even if you do hate it.

In order to make positive thinking yield results, you need to not only develop a positive attitude toward life, but also expect a successful outcome of whatever you do, and also take any necessary actions to ensure your success. For instance, you can't put your house up for sale and expect someone to buy it if you don't advertise or hire a real estate agent because no one will KNOW that it's for sale. If you hire a real estate agent who will advertise your home and bring people to see it, you know and can expect it to be sold.

Effective positive thinking that brings results is much more than just saying or thinking a few positive words, comments or thoughts. It has to be your predominant mental attitude. It is not enough to think positively for a few moments, and then let those negative thoughts enter your mind. Some effort and work are necessary. At first, it takes practice... after all, you are used to thinking negative thoughts, right? Habits are hard to break but if you are persistent and try to remember to think those positive thoughts after a negative one enters your mind, pretty soon your positive attitude will become your new habit.

WHAT IS POSITIVE THINKING?

Simply, positive thinking is the opposite of negative thinking. Positive thinking might take place in your mind, when you feel happy or when you have achieved something you have been wanting to achieve for a while. It's a little voice in your head (the one that's reading these words), that can put us in a more positive frame of mind on a day-to-day basis as we go about our lives.

Positive thinking is also one way a person can experience the feelings of positive emotions such as joy, happiness, excitement.

It may also put a smile on our faces and a bounce in our step, and make us look forward to things more.

Whether one has positive thoughts or negative thoughts, our minds are occupied with thoughts and depending on some factors, for some, positive thinking occurs more often than for others. But the great thing is that positive thinking is a skill that can be taught, learned, practiced and mastered such as you would be taught sports, practice music, learn a new language or master a subject.

Positive thinking can also become a Mind Set which is the next level of just having positive thoughts from time to time. A Positive Mind Set is such that the majority of your thoughts will be positive. And again for some people, the opposite may be true, but through proven steps, tools and practice, anyone can reprogram their mind to counteract negative thoughts and a negative mindset.

WHY POSITIVE THINKING?

Positive thinking is valuable to us in many ways. For example, if you're competing in a cross country or marathon event at a sports day, and you're running and running, feeling like your legs are going to collapse under you and your stitch will kill you,... you feel weak, muscles are melting, your lungs feel like they're going to burst and every step is agony. Like many top sports people do, they will use positive thinking to push through, not just to get over the finishing line, but to win. A positive mindset is also referred to as a "Winner's Mind Set".

And as we have established, positive thinking is the opposite of negative thinking. Negative thinking is the other voice or even other voices in our heads that might tell us we are stupid when we make mistakes or fail at something. Negative thinking can mentally paralyse some people too and stop us from asking for what we really want in our lives. For others, it might make them worry about things that may or may not happen.

With a positive mindset, you end up making better decisions, feel good and generally function better in life.

Positive thinking fuels positive energy which is a much higher and lighter energy than negative thinking and negative energy which is heavier and brings you down.

Imagine you are invited to go to a party or an event and you think negative thoughts such as,

"I won't go, no one will like me; I hate those people anyway"

Do you think you would be getting off to a good start to make new friends let alone a good impression? In fact you probably will end up not even going.

What if you went into it thinking

"How fun, new outfit!! I'll wear my new shoes!! All these new people I can get to know (or get to know me) I'm going to have so much fun!"

Which mindset do you think is going to end up having more energy and who do you think will actually go, stay and meet new friends at the party?

Positive thinking is not... about lying to yourself, or being fake. It's important to be realistic and truthful. Your brain will know if you aren't being authentic.

In order to begin thinking positive and living a life from a positive mindset, we have to start noticing positive things that occur all day long. This is being "conscious".

Being conscious is being aware of the thoughts you have, both positive and negative. It is also about noticing what's going on around you and how you internally react to these things and then translate and digest them into being positive or negative.

So to develop your positive thinking skills, beginning with being conscious is important. This is so you can really differentiate between negative and positive thoughts as they occur.

BENEFITS OF POSITIVE THINKING

It is common for us all to wake up feeling directionless every day. However, it is not the end of the world.

You must have heard people telling you to look at the bright side of life. So what is this bright side in real? Does it exist or do we need to create it ourselves? The truth be told, there is no bright or dark side of life.

If you master the art of thinking positively, you can jazz up your environment and always stay happy. Thinking positive has incredible benefits for us, but seldom do people try to keep away from thinking negatively in today's time. So, here are some mind-boggling benefits of thinking positive:

Increased Immunity

In the last few years, researchers have found that positive thinking has a concrete impact on your body. To stay fit and active, it is essential for your body to have a strong immunity system. If you continue to fall sick every few months up, it will have a strong impact on your mental and physical health. In one research, experts revealed that the negative energy released by the brain causes the immune system to get weakened.

Stress Relief

More than 500 million people across the world suffer from stress and anxiety, as a result of finances and work-related issues. When faced with such situations, even positive thinkers transit into pessimists.

In one study, researchers found that when optimists encounter a tough situation in life, they look for ways through which they can get rid of a problem. Rather than blaming everything around, they tend to carve a plan of action to get rid of the issue fast.

Believe in Your Abilities

Before you put on that white-colored hat on your head, keep in mind, positive thinking is not just about taking a simple approach in life. In many types of research, it has been found, positive thinking can help you for the rest of your life. For instance, over optimistic people often end up overlooking their inabilities in life, which later leads to stress and anxiety. So instead of overlooking reality, it is better to believe in your true abilities and continue to work on yourself.

Improved Wellness

No one can deny, mental health is related to the physical health of a person. If you're stressed out all the time, higher are the chances that you will engage in stomach related issues. Therefore, not only can positive thinking impact your ability to cope with anxiety, but also has an impact on the overall well-being of a person.

Although there is no concrete evidence that mental health benefits physical health, yet there are people who suggest positive thinking can lead to increased wellness. If you are always skeptical about life you can visit a tarot card reader, palmist or astrologer. These trusted tarot readers and astrologers help in predicting the future.

Better Resilience

If you don't know, resilience is the ability to cope with different problems. People who are resilient can easily cope up with mental or physical trauma. Instead of falling apart, such people tend to stay strong and cope with whatever calamity has befallen them.

It may come as a surprise to you, but positive thinking has a strong impact on enhancing resilience. When going through a challenge, optimists look for ways with which they can fix a problem.

POSITIVE THINKING: THE ESSENCE OF EXISTENCE

Positive thinking is a vibe that could easily fool the heart. At adverse times, when one thinks positive thoughts and acts on them, the mind could be controlled to relax and help see the big picture. People always assume that only the ones who are logical and have a practical or realistic approach to life succeed. But, that is not entirely true. Being logical or practical or realistic is important to succeed but staying positive and focused in equally important. A person with positive attitude and thoughts is said to have won half the battle even before it has begun.

This is clearly illustrated in the fact that Late Mr. Steve Jobs, who is the pillar behind Apple Inc. was at one point fired from his own company by a fellow colleague who he hired. But, he was not bogged down by this incident. Rather he was determined to take over the company again. He succeeded in becoming the CEO of Apple Inc. in a few years time and continued to be in the same position till his death recently. It was positive thinking with hard work and determination that helped him make Apple Inc. the company it is today. If Jobs had given way to negative thoughts we would have not seen the iPod and IPhone that are famous today.

Negativity in life drains out all the good things about a man. Positivity can change the life you are living and help you create your future that is more fulfilling and worth living. Everyone has a dream that is not lived because of the negative influence from people around us or taught by them. The worst of all is; most of the time people fail in life because they do not have the courage to live their dream fearing failure. One should build up an attitude that gives the perspective to look at failures as positive steps towards success. One should take measures to train the brain to look at failures as positive points that make them strong.

J.K. Rowling, the author of Harry Potter series of books did not turn rich overnight. She had to face 15 rejections of the first book before she was accepted to be published. She was a then recently divorced single mother who had no job and left without a penny. She had enough reasons to be a failure, but it was positive thinking and the ability to see the bigger picture in spite of the obstacle that has made her richer than the Queen of England.

Our brain is designed to give instructions on our day to day activities. It is our thought processes that have derived the formula and instructed the brain to dictate the actions. We are masters and we can always change the rules and ignore the nagging negative voice that has been put there by us over years of time. But, positive attitude is not something one can gain immediately. Negativity and pessimism are more like a disease that has to be cured over a period of time with effective training. Failures and negative feedbacks did not stop Thomas Edison from inventing many things which include the Light Bulb. He faced more than 1000 failures before he successful lit a bulb.

To develop positive thinking one must always make conscious choices and decisions and never allow pre-determined thoughts take the action course. The decision that one takes must focus only on the bigger picture. The mind is trained to believe certain things and ignore certain things as 'too good to be true'. Stephenie Meyer, a novelist who is famous for the Twilight series of books refused to publish them when friends asked her to do so because the story was good. Only after persuasion from a close friend she sent it to 15 literary houses to be ignored by 9 and rejected by 5. One agreed to publish and today she is reported to have made $40 million from this book series alone. It is true that if people around us can impact our thoughts and life in a negative way, they can do the same in a positive way too. Try and stay away from people who say you can't.

Seeing a bigger picture and creating a better future for yourself is difficult but not impossible. The secret recipe is, positive thinking.

Here are the four golden rules that you should remember day in and day out:

- Acknowledge the fact that you are a person with negative thinking and ready to change.
- Ignore all negative thoughts coming from within and negative words coming from people around you. Convert them as motivation factors and work on proving them wrong.
- There is no such thing as predetermined fate. Your fate and future is what you make or break.
- Nurture the creativeness from within and utilize the opportunities provided or create your own opportunities.

When building a positive mentality, you will face hurdles that you might and might not have control over. You should be aware of them and be ready to face them when you stumble upon them. Positive thinking will help you be successful not only in your professional life but also in your personal life because both go hand in hand. Most people fail in personal life because they failed in professional life and vice versa. But, that is not applicable to people who are believers. With positive thinking, you might not become a millionaire over night but, you will be happy and satisfied with what you have at the end of the day.

RULES OF THE POWER OF POSITIVE THINKING?

The power of positive thinking and the top ten rules in getting it is one of the hottest topic today.

This is because people are realizing that positive thinking and a positive attitude does affect life significantly. Have you heard of "The Secret" movie? It's rapidly making it's way around the world.

Whether you see a glass as half-empty or half-full can affect the way you treat yourself. We are in control of our lives and our destiny.

An idle brain, is a devils' workshop they say. This is not a positive quote. However, using this ideology in mind, we ventured to write on positive thinking, so that something productive would be achieved of our minds.

Here are the top Rules to Get the Power of Positive Thinking

Switch negativity around

Remove all negative thoughts by repelling it outright when something negative enters your personality. Channel that energy into positive thoughts. Positive quotes and positive affirmations will help to keep negativity away.

Be patient

Positive thinking is not immediate. You need to reprogram yourself in order to get remove any negative attitude you possess.

Remember that other people can sense your negativity

Before you do anything, be sure to have the right attitude. One reason why people fail is because others can sense their negative attitude and want no part of it. Positive thoughts, positive thinking, and positive affirmation create a positive attitude

Surround yourself with people who have a positive attitude

When you are engaged in an internal battle between your negative and positive self, you will need all the help you can get. Do not surround yourself with negative people who will just drag your positive attitude to the floor with their negativity.

Be healthy

All of the positive thinking in the world will not help you if you are six feet under, can it? You have to keep your body healthy in order to fuel your positive thinking. One step to achieving the power of positive thinking is looking after your body.

Pace yourself

You need to pace yourself in order to prevent yourself from collapsing. Take life one day at a time. Remember that you can not hurry into being positive. Be patient and you will achieve a positive attitude.

Be positive

Always look for something positive in everything new. When you encounter something unfamiliar, do not be afraid. Take a hard look at it and see it for the positive effects it brings, this will make your life easier.

Believe

You need to believe. You can not pretend to be a positive thinker. In positive thinking, you can not fake it because there is no one to pretend to. If somebody merely believes that you are a positive thinker, how can that benefit you? The most important of the ten rules of the power of positive thinking is that you yourself should believe it.

Be objective

This is very important in the ten rules for the power of positive thinking. Many people tend to see their lives for their failures and thus, they lose all hope of ever attaining in their goal. Some other people, filled with false pride, tend to magnify their success and they make all the wrong decisions.

Apply the change

The main characteristic of these ten rules of the power of positive thinking is the fact that they only bring you to the door. You have to open it yourself. Many individuals do not realize this, but we need these rules in order to appreciate life more. Some people think rules limit our achievements, but this is untrue. Without any rules, we would have been extinct centuries ago. Rules remove the chaos that is called life and impose sanity into it.

EGO: THE POSITIVE THINKING PITFALL

"Your imagination is your preview of life's coming attractions." Albert Einstein

Are you successful in your career field, in your family life, in health? Do you experience lack in one area or in all? Many of us are searching for answers online by visiting dating services, reading books such as this one, and maybe exploring work at home and other online business opportunities. WHY? Oh, I already know a hundred answers: to find love, to seek relief from health problems, to pay bills, to send the kids to college, to raise one's standard of living, to become wealthy. These are just a few and they are all good; however, everything in life manifests in measure according to the strength of a person's fears, wants, and beliefs.

A person can enter a garden and leave with a handful of tomatoes. He can go into the garden with a small basket and walk out with a lot more. One can enter with a bushel basket and carry home a bushel of vegetables. The point is, a person can't take home anymore than he or she is prepared to carry.

Today, most people are aware of what is commonly referred to as the Law of Attraction: think positively about something desired and it will come. Unfortunately, the opposite also works. Think negatively about something and those thoughts will create negative results. If one believes that he lacks ability his opportunities will be small and his bounty meager. If he believes he inherited health problems illness will be his dance partner. If one believes that he is worth only $500 a month that is all he will ever earn. If a person believes he is worth $10,000 a month he has prepared himself to earn that amount. A person can't go to the well and draw more water than his bucket, his beliefs, will hold.

There was a man who loved to quietly enjoy his coffee and newspaper, but his wife was a morning person and full of talk. He loved his wife but in the mornings for years he wished he didn't have to listen to her chatter. Little did he suspect that he was preparing himself to reap the consequences of uncontrolled thoughts. He didn't understand that we live in a garden where our wishes are always answered, a garden where everything we plant produces whether we unknowingly cultivate weeds or flowers.

Everything is energy; form is nothing more than consciousness made visible. Thoughts are things. We create them; they exist. Ripples on a lake move outward according to the energy generated by the penetration of some intrusive object. Thoughts do the same thing, both the positive and the negative. Sometimes the thoughts are powerful according to the emotion and belief behind them and they bring instant results, what some may call miracles; other times the thoughts build up results or form over time. The effect advances like a turtle, but come it does.

That was the case of the man who wanted silence. He got his wish. He slowly lost his hearing. Thoughts are not innocuous. They either create or destroy according to their positive or negative nature, and the immediate energy or constant repetition of thoughts behind them.

If one considers this premise honestly he or she can probably think of current situations and conditions that can obviously be tied to specific habits of thought, whether theirs or those of someone they know. How many people do you know who wear their 'condition' like a badge of achievement, the old woe is me trap? That is why fear is such a hazardous use of imagination. If a person fears failure more than he wants success, failure is what he will get. If he fears, believes, that he will never have enough money to travel he will never see Paris.

My point, it is all a matter of consciousness, as one thinks so shall it be, and that brings us back to the question, 'WHY'? Why do you want to earn money online, work at home, why do you want a spouse, or whatever you want in other areas of your life? Is your motivation selfless or selfish? Some men have always injured, destroyed, or even killed others for gold, for love, and for power.

They had strong egos and used the power of thought to realize their goals. Positive thought gurus abound; imagine it and it can be yours they preach. That is what I have been writing about too, but I left out one important consideration. Both negative and positive thinking produce; thoughts are cause and they produce effects.

Negative thinking doesn't just prevent one from achieving a goal. If positive thinking can take a person somewhere from zero to ten then negative thinking doesn't simply keep him at zero; negative thinking takes him somewhere between zero to minus ten.

Obviously then, one's mantra should be to think positively; however, there is a pitfall: positive thinking, when powered solely by the ego, cannot create perfection. The ego is selfish by nature. A man or woman can get rich, and achieve other goals, but at what cost to themselves and to others? If a person wants a promotion he can use positive thinking, but unchecked his thoughts may lead him to lie and cheat and in doing so, harm others and ultimately himself. Produce a cause and there will be an effect.

I believe that there is a Mystic Power that some call the subconscious, others the universal consciousness, and through the ages gods by various names. To use a Christian analogy let's call this power The Tree of Life, while its sister, the Tree of Knowledge of Good and Evil is an allusion to man's individual and collective egos. Eating the ego fruit destroys your garden. Weeds, negative conditions and events, will invade your crops. How many people have died or injured others while searching for Eldorado at the behest of their runaway ego? How many have reached the top stepping on the backs of innocents?

I believe that when a person can learn to want the same quality of life for everyone as he wants for himself, that man has created a portal of entry for the Mystic Power which will then guide that man and perfectly fulfill his every need with no negative attachments. You want to improve your quality of life, then want the same success for everyman, for your friends and family and for your rivals. The philosophy of loving one's enemies is not limited to the teachings of Jesus. Even though one may not physically harm another, wishing ill for that individual is cause, and when there is cause there will be an effect.

In the online world, there is tons of material about generating leads, leads, leads. Generate enough leads and a marketer will make money, but what about the people who, due to his actions, followed him into one online program or another. If he keeps climbing the ladder playing a numbers game, never looking back, never reaching down to pull up the person who followed him he is building a house on quicksand. One day his selfish 'grab all you can get by hook or by crook' thoughts will boomerang and come back as effects that bite him on the butt. Metaphorically speaking, he will lose his hearing.

It is my opinion that if a person truly wants to be successful in every sense of the word, in wealth, career, family, religion, and social areas he must cultivate this philosophy: "I Want that my every thought, my every word, and my every deed will be that which is best for all that is." With that as his guiding principle, no negatives will attach themselves to his plants like parasites. With that as his guiding principle he may come to understand that the real answer to my 'WHY' question is that what he really want is happiness, and with that realization he may find himself traveling in a completely different direction than he ever imagined. He will know that there is a Garden, and that it will be fruitful according to the measure of his thoughts.

WHEN IS POSITIVE THINKING ACTUALLY NEGATIVE?

And what are the steps you can take to practice healthy, balanced, positive thinking?

If you're a positive thinker, what does that mean, exactly? Does being positive suggest that you will only entertain positive thoughts? How could you possibly do that? Some people try, unsuccessfully, to do so. The reason for their difficulty in maintaining a so-called positive outlook is obvious.

Each day, an endless number of problems occur, and those problems demand solutions. But to find solutions, you have to consider the problems, and that seems to bring up a conflict in people whose goal is to be entirely positive. After all, you can't be aware of the need for a solution unless you're also aware of the problem. So unless you are avoiding all problems of any kind, you'll realistically have to think about problems quite often.

If it's common sense that to find a solution you have to look at the problem, then where did the idea come from that you should only notice the positive? It may come from a uniquely American idealistic tendency. It's worth exploring how this attitude -- that anything is possible if you're positive enough -- became both an asset and a liability that affects would-be positive thinkers everywhere.

This can-do spirit, when utilized appropriately, is associated with the confidence that lets you move forward, in spite of all apparent limitations. This can be a wonderful asset, at least when it gives you the strength to move forward amidst apparently challenging circumstances. Such positive attitudes have helped creative thinkers attempt bold projects that had never been attempted before, and have yielded great inventions, new styles of art, new businesses, and innovations of all kinds.

It's a shame that this bright side of positive thinking has become so tempting to so many people -- they fail to see the limitations that often surface when you're exclusively seeing only the good aspects of everything.

It's sobering to consider the shadow side of the can-do spirit. Consider the case of a company like Enron that refused to consider problems that their whistle-blowers were warning about. This can-do spirit, when combined with self-delusion, put the company in serious trouble, because they were so full of their own positive hot air that they considered themselves as beyond the need to listen to the warnings. Instead, they tried to escape into their own positive cloud of arrogant illusory assumptions about reality.

How a cheerful pop song encourages you to be in denial

The willingness to deny problems is strongly expressed in the popular Johnny Mercer lyrics of the Harold Arlen song, Accentuate The Positive. It was written after Johnny Mercer attended a sermon by Father Divine, who focused on the idea of eliminating the negative in your thinking, and focusing on the positive instead. In the context of a sermon, such ideas can be helpful and inspiring.

You go to a sermon to be lifted up, inspired, and given hope to face the upcoming week. And to those who were mired in the dark cloud o their own negativity, that message was probably perfect for helping to blow those heavy clouds away. Sermons have a useful purpose, and they also have their limitations when their emotionally charged enthusiasm is substituted for clear thinking.

Suppose that you do become entirely positive? Once you become inspired enough to get out of your own dark cloud, what happens when you shift to only letting yourself think happy and hopeful thoughts? There is a serious limitation with trying to cover over problems with exclusively positive thoughts. The happy talk makes you feel better for a moment, but it won't fix your problems -- they're still there. Unless you start looking at the situation and examining possible solutions, nothing will change.

When you look at the lyrics of the Accentuate The Positive song, the urge towards Denial is made plain, because you are urged to eliminate the negative. Now that seems, at first, to be a suggestion to avoid hopelessness. And ideally, maybe that is what the song is supposed to mean. If the song were suggesting that you can learn to be positive enough to consider creative solutions to your problems, this would be helpful.

Unfortunately, you can take the lyrics another way -- as a suggestion to avoid mentioning or thinking about problems. Many people take the meaning in just this way. Notice that immediately after the suggestion that you accentuate the positive, you are advised to eliminate the negative. Well, how will you interpret that suggestion? Ideally, you would eliminate the tendency to give up -- you would rise above hopeless attitudes. Properly understood, you would change your negative habit of thinking, and start looking for reasonable solutions to your situation.

However, many people take this line of the song, about eliminating the negative, as a suggestion to not bother thinking about issues, or dealing with problems at all. Such people tend to say that they are trying to stay positive. That often means that they don't want to look at problems at all -- also known as avoidance and denial. Such unwillingness to actively find solutions through honest assessment, while putting a gloss of positive spin on everything, actually leads to a downward spiral of disempowerment.

How well-intended metaphysical teachings contribute to denial, despair, and disempowerment

Metaphysical teachings seem to have contributed to this tendency towards denial, through simplistic teachings about the power of resonance. You may have heard that everything in the universe functions through resonance, where everything is compared to tuning forks that resonate with each other. Notice how this innocent belief, attempting to take a principle of physics, and use it as a metaphysical teaching, leads many people into the state of denial.

First, you are told that everything is resonating like a tuning fork. Then you are told that your positive thoughts are resonating with all the positive forces in the universe. And then you are admonished that your negative thoughts will resonate with all the negative forces in the universe.

How will you interpret that understanding? It all starts to sound serious and foreboding, and it brings up an irrational fear about discussing problems at all -- after all, they're negative, aren't they When you fear something, you try to avoid it. You may come to believe that looking at problems, or discussing concerns, is somehow amplifying a negative reality that will only make things worse.

Too often, the metaphysical teachings leave you with a modern version of the old-time fear of the devil. Except that now the modern fear is that if you look at a problem, or talk about concerns and issues in the world, that is somehow Negative and Bad, and must therefore be avoided entirely.

If only metaphysical teachings would share the fine points of how to utilize resonance in a balanced empowered way, that would be fine. They generally don't. Instead they provide the ingredients for fear and denial, where everyone has to agree that everything is fine, and that everything is magically getting better.

This used to be called sweeping things under the rug, and with extremist positive thinking, that lump in the rug gets bigger and bigger.

There are entire groups of metaphysical students who think it reasonable to only respond in conversation with positive agreement. They imagine themselves as contributing to a positive universe, and see every agreement and supportive statement as co-creating an ever-better world. If only it were so simple -- you could affirm your way to continual success in life, in a positive upward spiral of continually perfect improvement -- with never a mention about any problems.

Regrettably, this tendency to cover it over with happy talk leads to the opposite of happiness, because you feel gradually dissociated from reality, and disconnected from useful solutions.

Maybe this reminds you of the old saying, that if you don't have something nice to say, then don't say anything at all. Sounds suspiciously like disempowering denial, doesn't it? Does anything improve through this avoidance, or does a stuck situation just stay stuck?

The ever-positive style of possibility thinking has spilled into the business world, in which the upbeat, continually positive person is considered as helpful to the business, and the employee who scrutinizes the problems, or acts as a whistle-blower, is considered as a troublemaker to be shunned. Certainly there is a place for the upbeat personality, but positive spin and the can-do spirit can never replace clear thinking. And let's look at that phrase -- clear thinking -- for a moment.

Why neutrality and clarity have been wrongly judged as less effective than hyped-up happy thinking

Clarity is neutral, which is neither positive nor negative. And without clarity, you are either dazzled by the cloud of positive hopeful glitter in your mind, or brought down by the heavy clouds of despair. So this fear of hopelessness is somehow connected to the self-dazzled condition of puffed-up positive thinking.

Could it be that those who dogmatically insist that everyone should be positive at all times are actually harboring despair?

No wonder they have to be so positive all the time -- they fear that they will sink into a negative state. And they will, too, because they haven't found the middle way -- the state of clarity -- the path that transcends positive and negative thinking. Neutrality and clarity are neither positive nor negative, and so this frees you to see your problems in a calm, clear-headed way.

Where in modern thinking is the missing neutrality -- the needed clarity? Strangely enough, it shows up in the Johnny Mercer lyrics. After being told to accentuate the positive, and after being advised to eliminate the negative, you are warned not to mess with Mr. In-between. Ah ha -- it seems that Mr. In-between is the code word for that neutral state of mind that is neither positive nor negative.

But is it true what the song says -- that you must eliminate the in-between state? No wonder people think that they have to avoid that dreaded in-between state -- the realm of Mr. In-between -- so that they can enter the glorious land of the glittering positive state of mind.

But you weren't told about the wonderful, helpful aspects of in-between thinking, were you?

Whether in a spiritual sermon, or in a new age class, or in a business seminar, you were given the clear choice to be either positive or negative. That isn't fair to you, because most states of consciousness aren't positive or negative -- and they aren't supposed to be. Why is that?

Go beyond the limits of over-confident, naive thinking

When you look at a problem, you need to consider many possibilities for what the cause, or causes of the situation may be. You need neutral clarity for that.

When you consider possible solutions for the situation, you need to be able to verify those various solutions. You need to be able to consider the solutions with the clarity of mind that lets you recognize whether the solutions are appropriate and doable. Again, you re❑uire neutral clarity -- Mr. In-between.

What happens when you forget your neutral clarity?

Notice how when you replace your neutral clarity with simplistic positive thinking, your ability to scrutinize solutions becomes limited -- because all the solutions look great. Every idea is genius -- Not.

Likewise, when you get stuck in negative, hopeless thinking, your ability to find solutions is definitely limited -- because there is no room in the mind to consider solutions at all.

But why shouldn't positive thinking automatically give you the solutions -- after all, aren't positive energies supposed to inevitably lead in a positive direction?

The reason that positive thinking becomes negative is simple to understand, when you examine it for a moment. Positive thinking assumes that something is good, merely because you shower it with confidence and belief. And in real life, not all choices produce useful results -- and some can be dangerous. Positive thinking assumes that everything will work. In real life, that just isn't so. Positive thinking assumes that any choice, entered into in a positive frame of mind, is bound to be useful. This is not necessarily true.

Does this mean that if you let go of having to be positive all the time that you're giving up on positive thinking? Not at all -- you're giving up on extremism. You're giving up on denying your common sense. You're giving up on denying your intelligence. You're letting go of th positive thinking extremism that prohibits your right to calmly discover the solutions that are available to you -- when you are willing to access them.

So what is the proper place for the can-do spirit -- the anything-is-possible attitude -- the nothing-will-stop-us feeling? These are all designed to uplift your emotions. When you need an emotional lift, use these positive attitudes and feelings to lift yourself out of the swamps of hopelessness. But never assume that positive thinking is going to give you wisdom, common sense, or clear answers -- it's not designed to do that.

Properly used, positive thinking sweeps the cobwebs clear, and reminds you that solutions are possible -- but then, you will need neutral clarity to move forward effectively.

You need to be able to utilize positive thinking wisely, and you need to be able to use it for its intended purpose -- to keep you from getting stuck. But if you let yourself get locked into happy-talk land, where no problems exist, and where all solutions are equally good, then your condition is only slightly better than when you were stuck in negative thinking.

Guided meditation

This helps you access effective solutions with wisdom, clarity, and grace:

- Now consider the creative solutions. Just write them down in a list, even if them seem improbable, difficult, strange, or not typical solutions. Don't agree with them, and just get them written down.

- Now you're going to look over each possible solution -- the obvious ones, and the creative ones. Wear your clear-thinking neutrality hat.

- When you look at each solution, put that solution in a bubble of light. This keeps it in its own little universe, and keeps you from getting too attached to it. In this way, consider the obvious solutions, and the creative solutions. Write any insights you have about these.

- Look at a situation that concerns you.

- Imagine that you are containing that situation in its own bubble of energy. This gives you a bit of healthy distance, and lets you remain stable and centered.

- Here's where you get to be positive -- tell yourself that there are solutions for this situation. Don't start thinking about what they might be just yet -- simply know that solutions can be found. That's real positive thinking.

- Now put your positive thinking hat aside for a moment, and put on your clear-thinking neutrality hat. Imagine that you can look at the situation with a clear-thinking set of x-ray

spectacles, so that you can clearly look within the situation --
and you're still wearing your clear thinking neutrality hat.

- Look at the obvious solutions. Don't agree with them. Just write
  them down. Obvious solutions are the solutions that anyone
  would come up with. Just consider them, but don't align with
  them yet.

- Look over your notes. You're still wearing your clear thinking
  hat. If any of the solutions really seem inappropriate, cross
  them out of your list.

- Look at the possible solutions. While still staying fairly neutral,
  have a bit of a creative brainstorm with the ideas. Get a sense
  about which solutions are doable. Sense if you'd like to
  combine any of the solutions.

- In the coming days, explore -- in a sensible, grounded way --
  the ideas that seem most useful.

- If you find yourself getting into the dark cloud state, put on
  your positive thinking hat, and remind yourself that solutions
  are definitely available -- when you access them.

- And most of the time, you'll be wearing your clear thinking,
  neutrality hat. That's because you need to have a clear
  awareness of what's happening, so that you can move forward
  intelligently.

Clarity and neutrality -- the exciting new stars of higher awareness

If this idea of being clear-headed and neutral sounds boring, think again. Clarity is like turning up the magnifying lens on a magic microscope or telescope -- you can see the beauty of the heavens, or the deeper reality of anything you choose to examine, with exquisite clarity. Neutrality lets you be totally present. It's what the ancient sages were talking about when they told you to come out of your waking dream. They were always telling you to wake up, and now you have a sense of what that means.

Maybe it occurs to you that you can be positive and clear-headed at the same time. You can. The reason for suggesting that you put your positive hat aside for a time was so that you could get familiar with neutrality, and learn about what it can teach you. Positive expectations are all well and good, but when they interfere with your ability to have a clear sense of things, then you're indulging in something that is no longer positive -- ungrounded fantasy or denial.

Now you realize that you don't have to puff yourself up with continually positive happy talk. But, are there people who really are too negative? Of course -- they are the people who insist that there are no possible solutions, and that you have to just take life as it comes to you, since everything is futile. That's passive, hopeless, and negative. Don't get stuck there, either.

You aren't one of those negative people. More likely, you're reading this because you'd like to be more positive, but you had suspicions about whether positive thinking was the simple solution it's sometimes claimed to be. And now you realize that you can be positive in a healthy balanced way, because you have the means of being intelligently and sensibly positive.

There is a curious sameness about the world of the positive thinkers and the negative thinkers. The earthly waking dream of the negative thinkers, surrounded by their negative hopeless clouds, is not so different from the relentlessly positive thinkers who are puffed up with continual happy talk. Both types of people are stuck in a limited, waking dream that keeps them from the rich depth and clarity that life offers in each moment.

When you explore any situation without sugar-coating it with hyped-up positives, you have the means to confront the situation and discover creative solutions that really can make your life better.

Your life is endlessly fascinating -- not because you're pumped up with happy bubbles -- but because being present puts you in the front-row seat of the greatest event -- your own life. When you're present in each moment of your life, and you experience it with clarity, you realize that there is something more meaningful than dazzled happiness, and more fulfilling than a hazy hope for a miraculous fantasy future.

Welcome to this moment. Life awaits you, but it's here now -- not in a cloud of hope just down the road. Breathe into it now, let yourself look at any situation that deserves closer examination, and discover that the solutions are clearly there -- when you neutrally let yourself explore them.

POSITIVE THINKING TIPS

"Change of diet will not help a person who will not change his thoughts.

When a person makes his thoughts pure, he no longer desires impure food."

- As a Man Thinketh

All of us have many thoughts running through our heads all the time - both positive and negative. Positive thinking usually begets positive reality, while negative thinking usually begets negative outcomes. Both modes of thinking are in a constant tug of war in our minds, and the thoughts which dominate will be manifested in our actions and outlook. Positive thinkers tend to deal with life challenges confidently and are more likely to attain success than negative thinkers, who tend to look at everything non-constructively.

Obviously, we would prefer to put on our positive thinking cap most of the time, and leave out any room for negative thoughts. However, whether we like it or not, many thoughts keep running through our heads, including failure and other unhealthy pursuits. What we can do is to train our minds to focus on the good things rather than the bad, the happy moments rather than the sad, on what we have rather than what we don't have.

It is sometimes said that we will never really know what we have until it's gone. So, shall we wait for some things to disappear before we appreciate them? No, in fact, we can train our minds to focus on the brighter things in life, no matter how little they are, so that negative thoughts do not cloud our future outlook. Here are positive thinking tips to start cultivating a positive mindset:

Balance your desires.

We live in a place of opposites and duality - gain and loss, pleasure and pain, light and dark, male and female, love and hate. This is how life is. We can never have all the good things in life at the same time. In love, sometimes someone gets hurt. In wealth, there will always be people who are richer and poorer than you. Moderation is one primary key to happiness.

Be realistic.

Make sure that what you want is something possible. Hoping for something to happen which would never really materialize in real life will only bring you disappointment. For instance, you may wish to lose weight. Hence, you have to set a goal and act on appropriate measures within a period of time to achieve what you wish. No one can get slimmer overnight. Don't expect miracles or quick fixes, for they are seldom the real deal.

Learn from experiences.

Learning in a classroom is way different from learning in real life. In school, one learns the lesson first before taking an exam. In real life, one takes the test first before learning the lesson. The test in the real life is our experiences. If we failed in that test, i.e. the experience is not so good, we study the situation and learn the lesson. From here, we can avoid committing the same mistake twice.

Be detached from the outcome.

It is sometimes said that life is like a ferris wheel; sometimes, you're on the top, and sometimes at the bottom. There will inevitably be times in our lives where some things do not turn out according to how we plan or want. Do your best in important things, but don't be too upset if you do not get what you desire as some things are not meant to be. Don't be too attached on results alone, as this sole focus can only cause disappointments and upsets. Sometimes, it is the journey and experiences that can be valued and treasured.

Keep a list of your goals and actions.

Set goals you want to accomplish and map your plan to achieve them. When you are certain of what you want to do and carry out in your life, a stronger mind and will power will usually follow.

Keep your mind focused on important things.

Visualize fulfilling your goals. Develop a strategy for dealing with obstacles and problems. Concentrate on important things that need to be taken seriously, but at the same time, take time to relax and enjoy With a fresh and clear mind, there's a higher chance of success.

Start the day cheerfully.

How you greet the morning largely determines your outlook for th rest of the day. Welcome it with energy and high spirits, and chance are things will go okay and you can focus on achieving what you want

Ask for guidance.

Only God knows what lies ahead for us on a given day. He will surely appreciate a few minutes of prayer. Ask Him for guidance in your daily prayer. Have faith that He is more than willing to grant our requests as long as it is for our own good and in accordance with his Will. With God as our guide, it will be much less likely for negative thoughts to dominate our day. I can make it through this day. Nothing is impossible. After all, God is with me.

Try new things and challenges.

See learning and changes as opportunities rather than something to be feared. It is worthwhile to change attitudes and routines as long as they improve yourself and things around you. Doing new things could include considering more options for a project, meeting new people from different places, asking lots of questions. Through this, the flow of thinking is directed to improvement and negative thoughts are minimized.

Laugh. Enjoy and have fun.

Looking at the brighter side of life starts with entertainment and pleasure. Laughter is the best medicine, and that is very true in many cases. Whether you have a physical or emotional ailment, a few laughs and giggles can help alleviate some pain or lift heavy baggage such as anxiety, disappointment, or nervousness!

Associate with positive people.

In every classroom, work place, or simply anywhere you go, look for optimistic people and associate with them. There are lots of them, I'm sure. They can help you build self-confidence and self-esteem.

Be open.

We have to accept the fact that we don't know everything. And that we are continuously learning in every place we go, with people we meet every day. Our mind is so spacious that it is impossible to fill it up completely. Thus, we should open our minds to new experiences and knowledge that may help us become better people.

Plan the day ahead.

Minimize avoidable mistakes that will cause loss of productivity and negative results. Plan your work first, and then work your plan. Have clearly defined goals for today, in the medium and longer term too. You can refine your daily goals even before you get out of bed each day, so you can avoid firefighting issues that could have been avoided with proper thought and planning.

Love yourself.

Before you expect other people to love and adore you, you need to love yourself first. Make a positive commitment to improve yourself in learning, work, family, cultivating friendships, appreciating nature and pursuing worthwhile causes. Praise yourself as much as you praise others. When you start feeling confident about yourself, positive thoughts will naturally flow.

Know yourself.

There is no better person in the world who can tell who you really are. Know your passions, wants, likes and principles. Ensure you set aside some time each week for self-reflection in solitude. If you know yourself well, you will be aware of how far can you go physically, mentally, and emotionally.

Make it a habit to ask Questions.

This should likened with ignorance; rather, it should be associated with seeking more information to understanding matters more clearly. With more knowledge, comes more power.

Have trust in other people.

Although it may seem difficult and risky to trust anyone, having confidence in people is key to dispelling doubts and negative judgments. Develop a keen sense for identifying trustworthy people and associate with them. This will help you build harmonious relationships with your colleagues, friends and people around you.

Forgive.

Mistakes and failures are the root causes of negative thinking. If we somehow learn to let go of the pain, agony, and fear we try to keep inside, it will be easier to express our good intentions and reach out to other people. Forgive yourself and others for committing mistakes and the same time learn from them.

Count your blessings.

Focus on what you have rather than what you don't have. Focusing on our desires that do not materialize will only bring discontentment and disappointment that wastes our time. Instead, be thankful and appreciative with all the blessings we receive.

Leave your worries behind.

At the end of every day, before going to sleep, there is no need to keep bad experiences and unhappy moments that had happened in the day within you. Let them go, throw them out of the window and kiss them goodbye, and you'll have sweet dreams. As a new day unfolds, new hope arises. Keep believing and always have faith.

CONCLUSION

Being positive and have an open mind towards life is a wisdom gained through hard work and go a long way. But, once you master the technique of positive thinking, you can be happy and self sufficient even with a dollar in your pocket. Said and done, positive thinking never lets you down even if friends and family do in the hour of need. Give in yourself to positive thinking and you can live your life everyday unlike the people who die every day.

Printed in Great Britain
by Amazon

55004513R00027